RAW EXTREME MANIFESTO

WITHDRAWN

CHANGE YOUR BODY, CHANGE YOUR MIND, AND CHANGE THE WORLD WHILE SPENDING ALMOST NOTHING!

FRED HO

WITH

PETER LEW

PHOTOGRAPHS BY
RICK OCHOA

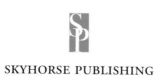

SKYHORSE PUBLISHING

Skyhorse Publishing books may be purchased in bulk at special discounts for sales promotion, corporate gifts, fund-raising, or educational purposes. Special editions can also be created to specifications. For details, contact the Special Sales Department, Skyhorse Publishing, 307 West 36th Street, 11th Floor, New York, NY 10018 or info@skyhorsepublishing.com.

Skyhorse® and Skyhorse Publishing® are registered trademarks of Skyhorse Publishing, Inc.®, a Delaware corporation.

www.skyhorsepublishing.com

10 9 8 7 6 5 4 3 2 1

Library of Congress Cataloging-in-Publication Data is available on file.

ISBN 978-1-61608-465-3

Printed in China.

CONTENTS

INTRODUCTION

After fighting colorectal cancer for four years and finding no solutions to beating cancer through the mainstream medical establishment, only more and more frustration, dissatisfaction, and mistrust fueled by institutionalized arrogance, I started on a different path of extremism to beat cancer once and for all without sacrificing my dignity, my quality of life, or my entire life savings.

This war against cancer, the unmitigated brutality of that war, along with the profound transformations fighting cancer has unexpectedly gifted me with (including new treatment modalities, new personal and philosophical paradigms, and the creation of the new Fred Ho) are told in real-time, graphic detail in the book *Diary of a Radical Cancer Warrior: Fighting Cancer and Capitalism at the Cellular Level.* One of the unexpected discoveries in struggling to defeat cancer was changing to a raw food diet, and the attendant benefits and transformations of such a commitment to raw extremism, to myself, and potentially to society and to the planet.

These changes (as I am discovering every second, experiencing the results at my cellular level), at first, promised to be extremely daunting. Many of my favorite and comforting foods were cooked. Could I give them up? Could I resist the temptations that we are bombarded with, from mouth-watering advertisements, to the seductively displayed cornucopia of exciting cooked items in stores and restaurants while I walked on city streets, to the meals eaten by my friends while I socialized with them? Could I really do this without cheating and compromise? Could I sustain this for the rest of my life, however long that may be, should cancer ultimately be victorious, which, according to the allopathicians (mainstream medical establishment), could be very soon if I, in their opinion, foolishly pursued anything other than their protocols and prescriptions (which are basically a paradigm of cut-burn-poison)? Would going to raw food work, help me beat cancer, or would it be, as the allopathicians viewed it, a foolish pursuit (because it had no clinical trials, no data; in other words, the studies have not been funded!)? Would I gain anything from going raw?

All of these doubts and anxieties did not hold me back from plunging into raw extremism. For my entire life, I have never been a person paralyzed by indecisiveness. I believe this attribute of decisive action is part of my warrior being, which began at a very early stage of my life from my many battles and struggles against racism, since the days of early childhood, to domestic violence growing up, to my entire adult life fighting for revolutionary social change in American society, to being an "avant-garde" artist working on the very fringes of the music business and nonprofit arts industrial complex, to the war against cancer in the past four-plus years. Part of this book is the why and how of becoming an extremist—how to internalize a combat-steel attitude of no compromise! Without this fortitude and determination, it is inevitable that we will succumb to temptation, return to bad habits and attitudes, not make the changes we need to make, and never fully move forward upon a new pathway of health, healing, and self-transformation—and create a new society.

I could not have gone raw extreme solely on my own, so I must thank my friend and comrade, Peter Lew, who cofounded the Raw Fight Club, a self-organized component of a revolutionary new project called the Scientific Soul Sessions (SSS) (www.scientificsoulsessions.com). Individual members of SSS interested in raw extremism formed the Raw Fight Club as a way to share information, to teach others the techniques of raw food making, to discuss and debate a range of topics including the U.S. medical system, the U.S. food industrial complex, capitalism, socialism, and our personal struggles. I drafted our Raw Fight Club rules, and we initially met weekly on Saturdays at my apartment and communally prepared and ate raw food dishes, sharing recipes and tips on the best ways to make the food, the benefits and changes we'd experienced, and mutual rants and scathing condemnations of the system of industrialized food production and medicine that we all believe is more harmful than healthful. Several of our members have rid themselves of chronic maladies that the mainstream medical industry has no solutions for, only "management" methods that invariably rely upon pharmaceuticals. In the case of our sister Ceci, for example, who eighteen years ago was diagnosed with multiple sclerosis and given no hope of ever walking again, here she is, in her mid-fifties, moving on her own two legs in her active life of organizing black urban farmers across the U.S.!

In this book, we make no pretenses of being nutritionists, doctors, or wellness workers. We are humble people with a range of educational backgrounds from all walks of life. The common dominator we share is that none of us is affluent, and most could be described as living either below or close to the poverty level in American society (I myself, due to my more than four years of disability as a result of the ongoing cancer war, subsist upon Social Security assistance, which is a little over $700 a month).

This is why this book is special and rare: our attitude and practices and goals are extreme and we are boldly proud of this; we believe that because we are extremists, we actually have solutions and dare to share our experimental, avant-garde beliefs and practices without any concern for mainstream acceptance and compromise. You'll never find anything like what is here in any other book, and most likely never will, until the revolution is well on its way to ending industrialism, restoring commonality and self-sufficiency, and replacing the capitalist system with something that eliminates the profit motive and its relentless pursuit and replaces it with ecosocialism (some of whose features and expressions are advocated and implemented in the contents of this book).

Our lessons and offerings affirm that health, happiness, creativity, weight loss, self-improvement, and social change must never be conflicted or contradictory, but rather holistic and synergistic, and that we can do it all by spending almost nothing (in terms of money, though time, effort, discipline, and creativity are required)!

This book conveys both my personal discoveries, as well as those of the members of the Raw Fight Club. Peter Lew has contributed large sections of this book. Remember, we are experimental, a perpetual work-in-progress. You may very well disagree with, oppose, or even reject our premises and assertions. We can't expect everyone who is trapped in the matrix to be any other way. It is a struggle, and the choice is yours. The journey will be difficult, and so the rules we've made for our Raw Fight Club are what they are.

We warn you that we don't sugar-coat anything (indeed, we are sugar-free!). But if you are seeking to make the personal and social changes necessary for health, happiness, and betterment, and can be open to extreme views and practices, in a short amount of time, we believe, you will find discoveries and improvements that will become persistent and irreversible. We know you will benefit greatly from this process and will be a new recruit for the raw extreme revolution.

Finally, I make no medical claims in this book. I, personally, am uncertain whether the changes I advocate herein will be sufficient for me to defeat cancer (indeed, I don't expect that any cure for cancer exists as long as global industrialized capitalism does). But I believe that what we do advocate and advise and show by example within these pages will greatly contribute toward optimizing health and prefiguring revolutionary possibilities for both individuals and society as a whole.

It is quite possible that no real "cures" on a societal level can be found to many of our modern maladies until we end the matrix (the mode of existence) that exponentially ensnares us in industrialized dependency. However, we are convinced and convicted believers that a mostly raw diet will offer tremendous preventative and palliative possibilities and is essential to any framework for wellness, both individual and societal.

FRED HO
BROOKLYN, N.Y., 2011

SIX RULES OF
RAW FIGHT CLUB

①

No compromise.

②

No compromise. If you compromise, you will be kicked out of Raw Fight Club.

③

Everyone must fight. No exceptions. If you're
new, you must fight first.

④

Anyone can join Raw Fight Club. Anyone can leave Raw Fight Club at any time.

You must talk about Raw Fight Club.

⑥

You must fight to win.

WHY GO RAW EXTREME?

After four years of mainstream medical treatments for stage IIIB colorectal cancer, I have had four tumors (two primary tumors with recurrences for each), seven surgeries (including a temporary ileostomy bag and its reversal, and for almost a year, constant ureter replacements for hydronephrosis of my left kidney that resulted from chemo-radiation toxicity), three bouts of chemotherapy that included all of the chemo drugs made to treat colorectal cancer (initially FOLFOX—fluorouracil, oxaliplatin, and leucovorin; and after that proved ineffective, then Xeloda, Erbitux and irinotecan), along with targeted radiation.

My trek through what I have called "the cancer war" included what many would consider to be the best hospitals in the U.S.: Long Island Jewish Medical Center (2006–2007), Beth Israel Medical Center (2007–2008), and the much-touted Memorial Sloan-Kettering Cancer Center (2009–2010). In the words of my friend and once-primary care physician, Dr. Joseph Harris, during those long, brutal four years, I was the "perfect cancer patient," disciplined, compliant, respectful, informed. But after the recurrence of a T3 rectal tumor (diagnosed mid-September 2010), fed up with the inability of mainstream (allopathic) medicine to provide any real solutions, I began to seriously consider a naturopathic treatment that would find a solution, and I vowed never again to return to the allopathic paradigm of more and more of the same treatments of cut-burn-poison (surgery-radiation-chemotherapy). I would find a solution and beat cancer, or I would simply die, but die with dignity and with no reduction to my quality of life until my expiration.

During the cancer war, for the first four years I had dismissed "alternative" medicine, skeptical of its efficacy because I could not find "evidence." Clinic trials or case studies were few and limited because, as I would later come to understand, pharmaceutical companies either saw no substantial profits to be made, or worse, opposed something that they could not patent that would empower the patient to become disinclined to rely upon drugs.

Examples of naturopathic successes were invariably anecdotal. Without being able to verify these anecdotes, to interrogate the patients who claimed to be cured, I remained wary and skeptical, especially at the prospect of risking my life with claims I could not interrogate and investigate.

This all changed when my friend and fellow activist Peter Lew introduced me to a stage IV metastatic colorectal cancer fighter, a thirty-something-year-old man who had done the allopathic treatments, suffered many losses, chose to reject any more such treatments, and had gone the naturopathic course, centering his recovery upon a very special raw food diet. This man, I shall call him Joseph, had become cancer-free, his tumors in his colon and liver, miraculously gone. I was able to speak to him for two hours, grilling him with questions, verifying his story, obtaining details on every aspect of his case and his methods.

He told me that he had converted to an all-raw food diet, which included eliminating all sugars (including from fruits and high sugar–producing vegetables such as carrots, beets, and corn), and in a year's time, had achieved what his allopathic doctors considered to be a miracle: he had beaten stage IV cancer after being given less than six months to live, even with radiation and chemo (including the dreaded super-drug, Avastin, which is considered a "miracle" drug not because it can cure stage IV colon cancer, but because it merely extends life for stage IV colon cancer patients on the average an additional six months!).

For the first time, I could verify that a naturopathic treatment had worked for someone. I didn't care if such "miracle" cases were a tiny fraction of the total—at least it was a solution that didn't entail more of the cut-burn-poison protocol.

My surgeon at the time at Memorial Sloan-Kettering, Dr. José Guillem, as well as the second-opinion surgeon I consulted, Dr. Joseph Martz at

Beth Israel Medical Center, both advocated that I have a complete rectal removal surgery and live with a permanent, irreversible colostomy bag.

I had had a temporary, reversible, ileostomy bag between tumors two and three for four months, and while I hated it, after the unremitting, horrific pain of the last surgery (for tumor three), which had led me to consider suicide, I was now willing to accept a permanent colostomy bag should it come to that. But now I wanted a solution, not to have my rectum completely removed, then live for whatever time I have left with a colostomy bag, and *still* have cancer return. When my sister, a mainstream doctor, asked Dr. Guillem what he thought my curative chances were if I followed the procedure he wanted, he smugly replied, "I don't know."

It was at that moment—the celebrated Memorial Sloan-Kettering surgeon, who had previously excised my T1 tumor, had no confidence in this new surgery for this recurrence, which had now become at T3 tumor—that I questioned why should I have any confidence in him or the procedure he wanted me to do.

It became clear to me that there were no longer any solutions to be found with mainstream medicine—that mainstream medicine, rather than aggressively focus upon solutions, focuses upon "managing" cancer and not truly curing it since such a cure requires an understanding of its causes, which I contend is the matrix of the teratogenic-carcinogenic-and-iatrogenic (capitalism being the cancer for the planet, the socioenvironmental toxicity of capitalism being cancer for the person, and the domination of profiteering in mainstream, as well as most alternative, medicine as making for the impossibility of a true cure or solution).

Like so many patients who discard the allopathic for the naturopathic, I now had nothing to lose. The allopathic options were simply more of the same, ironically, with no real guarantees for success.

Being in the cancer war for four years and encountering many other cancer patients, many of whom died either from worse or less severe cases than mine, I realized that the best and longest period of my "remission" was when I went to grow my own food on the organic farm of a friend in the northern Catskills. My friend's nine-acre farm, five acres of which were used for farming, was built in

1827, and for all those years it was kept within a family that raised and sold Christmas trees. The land had not been overtilled or saturated with chemical fertilizers and pesticides. It was naturally organic without being legally certified organic according to U.S. Department of Agriculture standards.

This farm grows all kinds of vegetables, including leafy, root, and fruit-bearing vegetables, as well as some fruits, such as melons and berries. Asian vegetables are also grown, including daikon radish, bok choy, and other Asian greens, as well as spring onions (scallions), onions, garlic, plenty of salad greens, celery root, squashes, herbs, five different kinds of basil, tomatoes, potatoes . . . about two hundred different kinds and types of edible plants. Combined with constant exercise, well water, fresh mountain air, waterfall and natural pond baths, sweat therapy and vitamin D from plenty of sunshine, and nutritionally dense food straight from the ground, I recovered in a matter of weeks and passed two colonoscopies. I attribute my improvement and temporary remission to this overall experience and especially to the significant improvement in my diet, which was, while I was working on the farm, overwhelmingly plant-based and high quality. I also attribute the recurrence of rectal cancer to the fact that for all of 2010 I did not go back to the farm and compromised my dietary ways by eating many more cooked foods and more industrialized and animal-based sources of protein. By mid-2010, I was eating ice cream and "regular" meals, which I enjoyed, gaining back weight and returning to about 220 pounds, conditions which encouraged the return of cancer.

After the institutional arrogance I experienced with Memorial Sloan-Kettering, I knew that I had to take command of my treatment, to find solutions on my own. I want to be absolutely clear that I am not advocating the naturopathic over the allopathic or making claims for any "cure"

from either, only that the journey to empower myself in the war against cancer led me to realizations, discoveries, and to creating a new Fred Ho (physically and philosophically) for which raw extremism was one important and beneficial by-product. Whether the benefits of raw extremism are primarily palliative, preventative, and wellness enhancing (including ending hypertension for myself and, for others, possible solutions to problems such as diabetes and heart disease) and not curative (against aggressive malignancies and maladies), the principles and practices outlined in this book, I contend, are essential and important to an overall program of individual and societal change that furthers health and self-sufficiency and challenges the matrix in profound ways in a struggle for the transformation of our existence, i.e., how and what we feed ourselves.

HOW TO GO RAW EXTREME

The commitment to go raw requires both the desire and discipline to do so, for which the first two to six weeks will be the most difficult. Our consciousness has been conditioned for years to only consider cooked foods because of their dominance and ubiquity in our modern, industrialized society. Furthermore, marketing, advertisement, and the ubiquity of all kinds of food vendors are all designed to entice, seduce, and ensnare us into not only eating the food presented to us but to also keep eating it, constantly and often, to our harm.

Obesity is the number one disease for American young people, and it is the fastest growing problem in newly industrializing countries such as China, where even a generation ago, the concept of fast food, cars, and processed foods were nonexistent. Industrial life produces greater sedentary lifestyles, for example driving instead of walking or riding a bicycle, or sitting in front of a computer or monitor all day instead of doing manual labor or, even more significantly, farming.

You will find yourself constantly fighting off the temptation to compromise, to rationalize buying and eating that small portion of your once comfort cooked food. How can you resist?

First, remove all processed foods and anything that needs to be cooked from your house immediately. You don't have to add to the mountain of garbage; take it to a soup kitchen or food donation drop-off center and give it away! In fact, learn to let go of a lot, not only material possessions but also emotional and psychological baggage, grudges, anger, etc. I have a rule: every holiday season, I review everything I own, and if I haven't used it within three years, I either sell it or give it away. Anything.

Once you start divesting your home of processed foods, you will find an empty freezer (since all frozen foods are processed unless you did it yourself) and an almost empty refrigerator. Your cupboards should also be almost empty except for a few dried herbs and spices, some oils (not used for cooking), and some condiments.

As soon as these are cleared, you can begin filling up with oils, raw nuts, dried seaweed, vegetable spices, and condiments. Once you are making delicious raw dishes, you can share these with the skeptics and the curious by putting what you make into those plastic containers, never asking for them back, and converting all of your storage devices to metal or glass. Recycled large glass jars with metal lids are the best storage containers. This costs no money. I keep a few plastic storage containers, but I really don't need them anymore.

Obviously, all processed foods have been removed and forever banned from not just your home but also your entire life, except for those which will be needed for your raw revolution. In many ways the supermarket, you will soon consciously understand, is superfluous. More on food sourcing later.

Second, and this is easier to do if you live alone or with people who are also joining the raw extreme revolution, turn off your stove and oven *permanently*! This is an act of commitment, of no return, of eliminating any possibility of compromise. For a gas stove and oven in New York City, this saves you a basic meter charge of $13 to $15 a month, plus whatever you burn. For the first period, avoid heating water (though later, should you want tea, you can get an electric tea kettle as discussed below). Just drink water.

There is a lot of controversy over tap water, especially the problem of dental fluorosis, irreversible staining of the teeth caused by overflouridation of public drinking water, a now acknowledged widespread problem, especially for young people. The problems posed by bottled water are also complicated and numerous, the least of which is the leaching of toxins from certain plastics and the enormous waste of disposing of all of those plastics (degraded plastic produces dioxin, a lethal toxin, which goes into soil and into water bodies).

The best thing is to live a plastic-free life. Plastics have only been around for and become ubiquitous during the past sixty years. Great cultures from all over the world have made do without plastics for several millennia and produced beautiful, efficient, and effective storage and conveyance containers and methods, including the Japanese bento box lunch, glassware, etc.

We advocate the elimination of plastics altogether and once and for all. Along with ending the internal combustion engine, a plethora of environmental stresses would be relieved, and such a commitment would reflect a determination to reverse the ecological disasters which modern capitalism has inflicted upon the earth.

After all, capitalism is the only man-made system in human history in which the existence of the ecology is exponentially threatened. Despite social classes, inequality, wars, and ruling class opulence of past civilizations, no precapitalist society had the potential to destroy the entire ecology of the earth as now-global capitalism threatens to do. This is why the topics of ecosocialism, deep ecology, permaculture, and other radical and revolutionary proposals for restructuring human relations both within our societies and with nature overall are critical. To think and act anything less than radically and revolutionarily is to perpetuate the problems of overaccumulation, overconsumption, waste, and expanding toxicity, and their myriad attendant problems, both for humans (such as the aforementioned obesity, cancer, and other maladies) and for every species of life that exists in our biosphere.

So for drinking water, which should be the sole beverage for the first phase of the raw conversion, if possible, glass bottles filled with well water from a friend's farm should be arranged. For one adult, filling a large recycled (yes, plastic) milk crate of gallon or large-glass bottles and jugs provides about two to three weeks of water supply. Another conveyance container to transport a collection of glass water vessels can be a sturdy crate with han-dles, though this will be heavier than the recycled plastic milk crate.

In many towns in other countries, including big cities, potable water from a local spring or well is very common. Human communities prior to the advent of the industrial city were located and built around such natural water sources. Today, people line up at these potable watering holes, though often with five-gallon plastic jugs. In cultures with advanced glassware craftsmanship, beautiful and durable octagonal water dispensers with solid brass spigots, in common in many Latin American societies, are a worthy purchase and, if bought while traveling in these countries, will cost a fraction of what would be paid if purchased in the U.S. I found one three-gallon glass dispenser with a solid brass spigot in a Salvation Army in the San Jose, California, area for $10, and it will last forever and is beautiful as well.

These premodern methods will be a constant template for a revolutionary transformation of our daily lives (even in this matrix!) as well as a precursory path to a revolutionary new ecocentric society.

So drink your water from a well, with all of its minerals and without the chemicals, though as long as global pollution, spill-off, and soil contamination continue as by-products of industrialism, water purity will be at risk.

Third, create and internalize psychological combat methods for yourself and for everyone else in the raw revolution. Here is a simple method I devised that works well for me. Part of figuring out what will work is to know oneself. The biggest affront and insult to me is to be called a *compromiser*. When I feel myself tempted or drifting, I mentally curse myself as a *compromiser* and my self-contempt for my weakness effectively dissuades me from the temptation.

When I walk and see food advertisements or displays that tempt me, I contemptuously curse these temptations with the epithet *industrial food*. I tell myself, "That's that industrial food crap." By calling it that, with an attitude of contempt, I am more easily repulsed and avert any weakness or compromise.

The greatest obstacle is oneself. If you are reading this book, you have shown a beginning interest to change. Change is never easy, always difficult. That is why when it is achieved, it is so rewarding. There are no magic pills, no easy answers, and no shortcuts. The great revolutionary Amilcar Cabral said: "Mask no difficulties, tell no lies, claim no easy victories." The raw extreme revolution requires sacrifice (of your past and problematic present), struggle (to change and go forward), and steadfastness (to not stray, compromise, deviate, or fail).

I often disgustingly hear from people whom I am trying to transform, "Well, I'll try." *Trying is lying*! You must do it, sure, one step at a time, but deliberately and decisively, with diligence and daily deeds instead of self-rationalizing excuses for incremental changes that essentially avoid doing the deeds needed.

Make no mistake: the raw extreme revolution is about the protracted struggle of making a revolution, simultaneously both internally (for yourself and your people) and for society. Neither comes first. Neither precludes or obviates the other. They are both critical, essential, and necessary in terms of conscious application at every second and with every fiber of one's being. It is about bringing into being a new being!

LOSING WEIGHT

Obesity and even being ten to twenty pounds overweight can generate many health problems, a number of which can be life-threatening. These include increased risks of heart disease; hypertension; joint, bone and muscle problems; sleep apnea; diabetes, etc.

As T. Colin Campbell's research and many published studies have asserted, a diet based upon animal sources of protein is statistically significant for increases in all kinds of diseases, including obesity, cancer, heart disease, diabetes, and other life-threatening problems. Conversely, disease rates significantly decrease for people who eat plant-based sources for the majority of their food consumption.

I also want to stress that the primary pursuit should not be losing weight but gaining health. Weight loss should be a consequence of, as well as a means to, gaining greater health, vitality, and self-satisfaction. In going raw extreme, dieting and diet plans are meaningless and irrelevant. Weight loss will be a natural consequence of eating what we all should and must eat, and that is from plant-based sources. Raw extremism is not only converting to plant-based diets, but also a journey and commitment to fundamentally change food production, and activism toward a new and different form of human society altogether. All of these transformations require ending obesity: for our bodies and for the overconsumption and waste produced by a social matrix of consumerism, acquisitiveness, and the inexorable accumulation of capital and its attendant industrialism. Shedding excess body fat and weight is part of shedding our obese obsession with things and money.

Going raw and raw extreme, more than going vegan or vegetarian, is the surest, quickest, and most effective path to permanent weight loss that is irreversible. The popular joke is that French fries are "vegetables" and can qualify to be vegan-acceptable.

Vegan, macrobiotic, and vegetarian diets are all marked improvements, both for individual health and social change. We advocate rawism as a more revolutionary approach with, we believe, more revolutionary results.

A raw diet can include raw seafood. Indeed, anything from the sea that can be eaten cooked is also edible and, perhaps more enjoyable, raw! The only caveat to seafood, especially with fish which are highest or higher up the oceanic food chain (such as salmon, tuna, and swordfish), is the increased mercury content from the increasing contamination of our world's oceans from industrial pollution and waste dumping.

I remember snorkeling with my friends Richard and Mark Hamasaki in Oahu (Hawaii) and at-the-time young sons (Napu and Kai) and using metal tongs to pull out spiny sea urchins embedded between rocks, scraping them on scraggy rocks on shore or in shallower waters, and once de-needled, cutting open their encasements and feasting on the soft, tasty flesh. Sea urchin (which is called *uni* in Japanese sushi and sashimi) was a major delicacy for the royalty of *Ka Pae 'aina*—the traditional name for the kingdom of what the U.S. has called Hawaii.

You will easily lose weight once you begin going raw. The raw extreme path requires that you eliminate all sugars, including natural sugars from all fruits, dried fruit, and high-sugar content vegetables (such as beets, carrots, tomatoes, and corn). Green leafy and cruciferous vegetables (vegetables of the mustard family, especially mustard greens, various cabbages, broccoli, cauliflower, brussels sprouts) should be the mainstay of a raw extreme meal, along with raw nuts. After fast weight loss has begun, in approximately two to six weeks, adding certain "sugary" vegetables and fruits will be fine.

Juicing green leafy and cruciferous vegetables, adding as you like raw ginger, cucumbers, parsley, and whatever you might find appetizing and invigorating, should also be done daily. Usually juicing is done in the morning, sometimes in lieu of breakfast, with aggressive hydration, including water and tea.

Again, once the raw diet becomes easy and the results and changes to your mentality, physical being, and way of life occur, you can add natural sugars including fruits, honey, maple syrup, high-sugar vegetables, etc.

Always make sure you hydrate well during the day. Your main hydration source should be water, preferably well water. Lacking well water, then use either filtered water or alkaline water. Get rid of all plastics, including containers. You can carry your water with you easily in a glass bottle; sew a simple carry bag for it or make a rubber O-ring attachment of nylon strap (easily recycled from a bag strap) or, if you are fancier, a leather strip that either has a snap clasp or a simple key ring clasp that can clip onto your pant belt loops, your carrying bag, backpack, or luggage.

Continue all of the other healthy weight loss requirements: physical activity, exercise (cardio and strength-building resistance, neither of which require gym memberships or fancy equipment, yoga or stretching, daily and constant deep inhalation breathing, and meditation.

With this simple daily change of routine and lifestyle, you don't have to count calories, step on a scale, or worry about nutrition or portions. You can eat huge amounts of raw food and still experience steady weight loss.

But if you were overweight or heavy to begin with, you should do extra resistance exercise; manual labor such as farm work is an additional benefit for a new, transformed person who grows his/

her own food and gets plenty of exercise from that work.

Walking or riding a bicycle to where you have to go is best, though suburban living, discussed below, is fraught with a multitude of personal health, societal, and ecological problems, beginning with the dependency upon the automobile to get around.

Create many opportunities for communal and social meals with fellow raw foodists and talk trash about industrial food and your past lives; talk big about visions of social transformation that lead to the elimination of mass production and all of its by-products and entrapments. You'll have plenty of laughs while enhancing your consciousness and commitment! This is no compromise, no return—just crack plenty of jokes and share abundant laughter while increasing knowledge and self- and societal change.

In four weeks, I lost forty pounds as my body was frenetically burning all of my fat while being fed with powerful nutrients. But the key was eliminating all sugars, carbs, and starches in the initial period. Note that I didn't say fats. Extra virgin olive oil, flaxseed oil, grape seed oil, sesame seed oil—these all have no trans fats and, when not cooked (as in frying and, worse, deep-frying) not only retain their robust and pristine flavor, but pose significantly fewer potential coronary risks.

By losing weight, dramatic health improvements will soon become apparent and permanent, including lower blood pressure, elimination of diabetes, better sleep, increased stamina, breathing improvements, reduced problems with heart disease and high cholesterol, and even possibly diminishment of cancer tumors.

Your stomach will shrink dramatically, and problems with oversized meal portions will become irrelevant. You'll eat until you feel satisfied and full. You can graze during the day. I have a large glass jar of mixed nuts or plenty of avocadoes or crudités for snacking and freshly-made almond drink, and after losing over thirty pounds and feeling sure I was not going to compromise or return to the past ways, I added dried fruits, including delicious dates and figs, and a sparse amount of fruits and fruit juices. I will never again buy premade, processed juices of any kind, which, as one grocer in the produce section remarked to me, is, after all, mostly sugar. (Ever notice that fresh-squeezed orange juice is "lighter" and more delicious than Tropicana or processed juices, and leaves your thirst quenched, while processed fruit juices always have an acidic and gritty aftertaste?)

There are also other ancillary, yet important, lifestyle changes. Get off the computer, stop text messaging, and eliminate sedentary fixations with electronic monitors, including Kindle! Go for walks, work in gardens, devise new exercise activities, walk or ride a bike to the library or used bookstore simply to browse, practice a musical instrument, make love, play with your kids or your friends' children, and always teach by being the example to all.

In my north Brooklyn neighborhood, even in the worst weather, I always have a mile walk—stopping in at my favorite places (including secondhand stores), just seeing what's around, noticing *existence*.

As your body increases its metabolism, burning off fat and restoring energy and stamina, you should respond by increasing your activity toward the raw revolution through voluntarism, organizing, noninstitutional education and arts, and planting and growing food, thereby constantly challenging the status quo and any possibility of compromising and faltering.

Four weeks after I started on the raw extreme path, my waistline shrank from 42–44 inches to 35–36 inches; my clothing, once XL to XXL, is now M to L; my shirt neck size, once 17½ inches, is now 16½ inches; and I can do more push-ups and chin-ups, and swim faster and longer than ever in my entire life. I brag that at age fifty-three (at the time of this writing), I am in better shape than when I was twenty-three!

Without losing strength and muscle tone, but with major weight loss, I have exceeded my personal bests in my regular isometric workout, and I'm not exercising any more than I did pre-raw!

Finally, even according to mainstream advocates of weight loss and better health, eating late-night meals can produce a host of problems, especially weight gain. I advocate not eating any meal after 7 PM at the latest, and if you are hungry, either graze (with raw nuts and possibly dried fruits) or bite the bullet and experience what most of the world experiences: going to bed hungry. There is no better way to self-instruct humility and self-control and understand the sharp contradiction between obesity in affluent societies and poverty-created hunger for most of the world's population. There is nothing wrong with going to bed hungry in the U.S. when it is self-imposed and not a consequence of extreme poverty and financial hardship, but rather, acquiring asceticism, humility, empathy, and curing obesity.

DRINKING WATER AND FRESH-SQUEEZED GREEN JUICES

Without any alcoholic drinks or processed juices, and initially with no fresh-squeezed fruit juices, all of the extreme changes occurred rapidly. I continue to drink mostly well water, tea, almond drink (see recipe chapter), and fresh-squeezed green and cruciferous juice. I have no desire for sodas, coffee, or processed drinks of any kind. I also don't even purchase store-prepared, so-called fresh juices since I prefer local and organic sourcing, and why spend money when I can easily and enjoyably do it myself?

On the topic of water, all sorts of expensive water sourcing is commercially available, from bottled water (of all kinds and purported health benefits) to alkalinized and ozonated water machines.

However, all of these much more expensive methods don't provide any more benefits than what we suggest below.

I have friends who have a residence in the northern Catskills that they visit most weekends. They are a married couple with two children. The wife has been fighting throat and face cancer for more than twelve years, and we give each other mutual support and share information, and she brings me back large glass jars and jugs of her well water, about ten to fifteen gallons, which takes me about two to three weeks to drink. I use filtered tap water to make tea or soak my raw almonds and make almond milk. I prefer to save the well water solely for when I just want to drink water.

Additional glass bottles and jars are easily procured from recycle bins in my apartment building or from friends.

There are two basic kinds of juicers. One is centrifugal, high speed, the best of which have a large vertical or top opening, or mouth, to "feed" the fruits and vegetables to be juiced. The others are side-fed and operate at slower speeds, which reduces the heat friction and gives more robust juice, especially from delicate leafy greens (such as spinach). The latter are about double the price of high-speed juicers. Wheatgrass stainless steel hand-cranked juicers that don't require electricity and are excellent tools also provide the benefits of a good upper-body exercise as you really have to use your arm muscles to keep cranking the extracted juice from the wheatgrass.

Growing wheatgrass is something that, while simple and easy, requires experience to do well. Wheatgrass is available through a number of wheatgrass-juicing kits and online and through book sources. Wheatgrass is heralded for being "the perfect liquid food" and "complete nutritional source." Because of its intensity, it is hard to consume more than a small amount at a time, so growing a modest amount daily is no more difficult than tending to houseplants on a regular basis. The challenge is to never overwater and to have good drainage, otherwise the wheatgrass tends to drown easily.

Chlorophyll, both as a source of hydration and oxygenation, has been claimed to further antiaging and produce a myriad of health benefits. Again, we are not scientists and doctors and cannot confirm or deny such claims. However, as a source of fiber and nutritional enhancement, we believe that green juicing, directly done and not processed, is part of disengagement from industrial dependency and is both health-promoting and a delicious and invigorating food source.

THE REVOLUTIONARY CORNERSTONE: FOOD SOURCING AND HOW SELF-IMPROVEMENT AND CHANGING THE WORLD HAPPENS

As discussed earlier, self-improvement requires never compromising principles, the discipline and commitment to seek total, as opposed to partial or piecemeal, transformation, and to go "beyond the beyond" (ultimately, to achieve results and outcomes that you could never have imagined and I bet most others, especially those in the mainstream nutrition and medical fields, couldn't prescribe much less even expect). Losing fifty-five pounds in about four months of time without sacrificing the quality of my life, including the quality of my food (but, rather, improving that) . . . who would've thunk? I never did, nor did my friends or family and, certainly, no professional trainer, nutrition therapist, or professional would have prescribed, much less believed, that I could have done this, and most importantly, done this on my own *without* their professional help (i.e., by paying them!).

I am not a well-to-do person financially. For all of my adult life, I have been a struggling avant-garde artist and, as you can read in these pages, a flaming, radical extremist! Now, I have done fairly well considering most composer-musicians aren't able to make a full-time living from their art, much less such a living without compromise and by only doing the art that they want to do. Most who are successful in the arts, if they weren't fortunate to become stars, have had to do "work for hire" employment, usually as side people or free-lance performers, commercial gigs (weddings, jingles, staff assignments), etc.

In the four-plus years of fighting advanced colorectal cancer, I have not been as financially gainful as I was in the past, which was still pretty low. I never made more than $37,500 a year net. Since the war against cancer, I've had to live off of federal Social Security disability and my savings, along with some assistance from family and friends.

Even when I was working full-time as a producer-composer-band leader-musician, I was very frugal and careful with expenses, and had no embarrassment about buying from thrift stores and bartering or negotiating.

Here are some simple changes that take almost no, or very little, money but will reap tremendous benefits and spur pathways to societal change, especially in eventually making irrelevant the industrial system of mass production and replacing it with greater self-sufficiency and cooperative relations, thereby enhancing self and community symbiosis.

GO SECONDHAND

Many thrift shops, such as Salvation Army or Goodwill, flea markets, and yard sales have an abundance of items that are needed to sustain the raw extremist. Juicers, blenders, food processors, bowls, utensils, etc., are easily found at these vendors, and the less formally retail they are, the more possibility for price negotiations.

Should you be traveling to other countries, huge public flea markets and many self-help, non-governmental organizations (charities) have secondhand stores where your purchases go to worthy causes. In New York City, Housing Works is such a local chain of secondhand, "gently-used" merchandise of extraordinary high quality at a fraction of the original price. An entire comfortable lifestyle could be easily sustained simply from the throwaway belongings of the wealthy. Get that going. On my daily walks, I pass by at least two secondhand stores, and I walk through them and see what I find for a bargain.

I have given away just about all of my plastics in my kitchen and replaced them with glass, ceramic, brass, metal, and wood containers. It is not important to have perfectly matching items; indeed, my aesthetic is much more eclectic and interesting than boring uniformity.

My friend Peter Lew found a fantastic nine-shelf dehydrator, for one-third the cost of brand-new retail one, at a secondhand store, with which he has made batches of delicious dehydrated kale chips.

Also, you can put out gift lists for holidays, your birthday, or, in my case, for when people learned of my fight against cancer and wondered how they could help, especially friends from far away. I asked a well-to-do couple, my friends Woody and Netta Igou, to purchase and ship me a dehydrator and a wheatgrass start-up kit with a stainless steel wheatgrass manual juicer. They were more than eager to help, and I am more than appreciative of their generosity and kindness.

By going completely raw, you'll find a lot of cooking gadgets and gear unnecessary and irrelevant. You can sell these or exchange them for what you do need.

RAW SOURCING

I go to my local organic restaurant, EAT (www.eatgreenpoint.com), and exchange cookware I no longer need or use for (raw only) meals or vegetables because I'm a friend of the owner and an ardent supporter of his concept and mission of healthful, local, and organic vegetarian food.

The problem with sourcing raw food (through either restaurants or markets) is the tremendous cost that is the disease of what I call "raw chic." When celebrities and pop culture stars take up any lifestyle change, hype seems to be the attendant disease, spreading like a cancer, driving up prices. This gentrification of raw, making it hip and trendy, has crazily driven up prices for something that is actually cheaper than industrial, cooked food simply due to the fact that less labor, fewer materials, less cleaning, and less industrialism is what the raw extreme revolution should be about.

The "industrializing" of raw food is making raw dishes that are "just like" cooked dishes, just as the fake meat/soy protein craze appeals to people who want something "just like" steaks and burgers. So at fancy, pricey raw food restaurants, the menu offers items "just like" burritos, burgers, etc.

The solution for the person and the planet is to be part of growing food on one's own and/or working cooperatively doing so. I currently don't own my own farm or urban food garden. But I have found friends who do and I go there as often as I can, which, during the growing months of April to October in the U.S. Northeast region, is usually one week out of every month during this season. In exchange for my labor and free saxophone lessons, which I give to my farmer friend Tovey Halleck, I get a bushel of vegetables and berries for every week during the season. I stay at his farmhouse and need very little. I work about five hours a day (he works longer as he is younger and also not fighting cancer). The benefits to us both are enormous and incalculable.

Here's what he gets: my diligent labor (I'm no slacker), which is a lot and which is important to him as he really has no farmhands or employees to work five of nine acres which he grows on, and free saxophone lessons from a world-class artist, and any questions he has about music answered.

Here's what I get: country fresh air, vitamin D from ample sunlight, fresh well water to drink, exercise without paying for a gym membership, sweat therapy (ridding toxins from the pores of my skin by sweating them out of my body), and unlimited, straight-from-the-ground, organic food which I often eat raw, snacking while I'm weeding and planting. I may cook a meal for Tovey (he isn't a raw foodist) while I just eat the fantastically delicious and high-density nutritious plants, usually plain without anything except for some oil and Bragg apple cider vinegar for salad dressing. I go to sleep shortly after sunset, sleep soundly, and awake totally refreshed.

And no money is ever exchanged. I get to his farm by hitching a ride with him during the week I'm going there. When he comes into the city to make deliveries of his produce to restaurants, we meet and I ride back to his farm with him. I return to the city when he returns to make deliveries the next week.

In this completely bartered exchange, the monetary nexus and all of its potential friction is completely absent. We have deepened our friendship and mutual respect, and taught each other a lot about things we never expected to learn.

You may say, *I don't know any friends who own farms or are farmers.* But some of the friends you do know may have a plot of land or a potential rooftop garden or may be interested in collectively getting a food garden started. The effort to make this happen is the first process of one's extrication from the industrial matrix. As you grow organic, especially avoiding the burden of organic certification if you aren't growing food for sale but for self-consumption, you avoid many of the by-products and problems of industrialism such as pesticides, fertilizer, machinery, employees, certification, regulation, taxation, etc.

Composting communities, recycling tools, containers, getting in-kind donations: these are some of the many ways to become deindustrialized, more communal and on the path to self-sufficiency, collective health, community building, commons restoration, and naturopathic consciousness—all necessary and critical components to an ecocentric revolution.

Mel Bartholomew's book *Square Foot Gardening* is exemplary as a model for nonindustrial urban food cultivation. Mel asserts that a four-by-four foot garden plot is all that is needed to grow enough food year-round to sustain the needs of two adults. An entire urban population's food needs could be met from the urban land that is either unused, abandoned, or misused for malls, parking lots, sidewalks, parks, etc.

An easy, convenient sourcing method is to join a local CSA (Community Supported Agriculture) program. There are many types. Some require a membership or that you purchase shares (like a co-op) for a period of time, which entitles you to regular supplies of what is local and seasonal. Others are simple pay and carry: you show up at a regular day and time during the season and either buy a prepicked container or choose and pick as you go. Often these are at farmers' markets or retail days at a local farm (commonly at the end of a work week). With the fixed boxes or containers, you usually don't have a say in what is available or in the quantities.

LIVING ALONE VS. LIVING WITH A LARGER HOUSEHOLD (THE CHALLENGES OF AND PROPOSALS FOR CHILDREN)

I have never been married (it's not something I have ever wanted) and have never had children (nor do I think I will desire any—though I have biological and nonbiological nieces and nephews).

It is much simpler to make profound and fast changes if one lives alone and has only one's own life to be responsible for. Many more complications and challenges exist for those with larger households (nuclear and nonnuclear family arrangements), especially when these members have been inculcated into the industrialized status quo of processed and cooked foods, shopping, consumerism, etc. Neither Peter Lew nor myself have any experience raising families of any kind. However, though we both are single men, we are serious and committed about building community and a larger movement for fundamental social change.

The process of going raw extreme requires constant discussion and leadership by example. No amount of didacticism, lecturing, self-righteous, or imperious attitude will work. Patience and daily effort at figuring out how to transform one's consciousness and practices will be the key, as it always is in any effort to effect real and substantial change.

However, I have spoken to and shared much of my raw extremism with many young people from ages six to young adult teenagers (nineteen years old), all of whom have shown interest and excitement, albeit perhaps slowly wanting to engage and pursue this path. The best leadership is always by example. Communally making raw dishes (see many of the recipes provided in the next chapter) is fun, educational, and engaging. Also, the extremism of turning off one's stove and oven *permanently* is an adventure and almost instantaneously drives many profound lifestyle changes that, when combined with farming and new sourcing activities for water and kitchenware, generates immediate excitement and instant change. Of course, openness to change and continual commitment to that change is a steadfast and constant challenge.

The process itself offers deeper relations among people, intentional aims at new goals based upon social change prerogatives, and personal and societal improvements that each person is an active participant in and contributor toward.

But the desire to become self-sufficient, to extricate from the industrial matrix, and to change one's mind, body, and role in society must be the primary and principal motivation, rather than a trendy fashion-following of "going green" or "localism," all the while spending more money and buying into the "chic" factor of capitalist consumerism and dependency. The goal is to become independent social beings who devise solutions and practical methods that are daily practiced, organized, and promoted to others.

The Raw Fight Club was the nucleus of our raw extreme movement, but everyone can creatively construct their own clubs and self-organizing examples.

Just having conversations about the importance and benefits of raw to the person and to society initiates that rippling effect. When the examples are presented, such as at a social event for which the meal is all raw combined with great cultural and educational presentations, the raw extreme infection is spread. For example, my Afro Asian Scientific Soul Duo, featuring myself on baritone sax and my longtime friend and colleague Dr. Salim Washington, performed at an event organized by the Independent Media Sanctuary in Troy, New York. The concert and lecture presentation Salim and I gave was followed by a raw food reception organized and hosted by raw food proponents locally, which supplemented our respective talks about how Salim and I went raw and its meaning and significance to our revolutionary musical, political, and personal visions. People had a great time in the concert, postperformance talk-back, and during the reception. It was an example of social change activism and engagement that was holistic and synergistic, combining music, political discussion, and raw food production and participation.

Whether going raw involves children and/or other adults, the activities can be organized and practiced in fun, educational, and transformative ways. Making a "shopping list" of secondhand cookware items (such as a food processor, dehydrator, glass water urns, jars, and bottles, wooden utensils, etc.) can be shared, and searching through the many secondhand stores, flea markets, and tag sales can be a lot of fun and very rewarding, especially in terms of great bargains and huge amounts of money that are immediately saved.

One favorite activity we have found with children, especially, has been making dehydrated kale chips because they are so easy and fun to do without any danger of potentially being burned by hot cooking oil used in making cooked chips or French fries. Kale chips are never greasy, very nutritious, and very addictive in their taste and flavor. These are the chips you never ever have to fear will make your children obese.

You'll also enjoy having a lot less cleanup, especially the lack of grease and grime from baking and roasting meats.

Introducing raw food at potlucks and events adds an interesting and, to many non-raw foodists, an "exotic" quality to the gathering, all of which is potential for further discussion of the raw extreme revolution, its personal health benefits, and a larger, more comprehensive vision of social and environmental responsibility and transformation.

But the strongest and loudest example is the change in you! Not only will you lose weight and be healthier and more energetic, which has many attendant psychological and spiritual benefits to enhance self-confidence and self-esteem, but you will be actually living the social change you espouse. And the raw extreme revolution will be taking root and flowering.

RAW EXTREME RECIPES
FROM A TO Z

ALOO PALEEK

This dish is very hearty and warming and goes well with our dahl (page 99). Lacinato kale is one of your best friends. Eat or juice it whenever possible.

Ingredients

1 bunch lacinato kale
3 cup walnuts
1/4 cup lemon juice
pulp of 1 Thai coconut
1/4 cup coconut water from
    above coconut

3 tsp Celtic Sea Salt
3 tsp cumin
1 tsp kalonji
1 clove garlic

Directions

1. Soak walnuts for 1 hour.
2. While walnuts soak, de-stem kale and cut into strips.
3. Massage salt for 9 or 10 breaths into kale strips.
4. Grate garlic with a fine microplane grater.
5. Drain water from walnuts.
6. Blend all ingredients except kale in a blender.
7. Mix all ingredients in a bowl and serve.

BAECHU KIMCHI

Kimchi is Korea's national dish, eaten with every meal as a side dish. Baechu is the traditional, most popular form of kimchi, with napa cabbage as the base. Fermentation serves several purposes. First, it is a traditional way of preserving vegetables in preindustrial societies. In Korea, autumn begins the preparations for the long winters, and kimchi making is in full swing following harvest. Second, it provides a variety of probiotics and enzymes that make this a very potent food, literally alive with beneficial microorganisms. It is one of the best foods for the gastrointestinal tract, the heart of the raw diet. There are many varieties of kimchi. According to the Kimchi Museum located in Seoul, South Korea, they number around 180 and growing. Experiment with fermentation time, as it is a process based on ambient temperature and personal taste. The brine can also be used as a drink or soup base.

Time Frame: 1 week

Ingredients (for 1 qt)

4 tbsp sea salt
1 head napa cabbage
1 daikon radish
1 or 2 carrots
1 or 2 onions and/or leeks
and/or scallions and/or
shallots (or more)

3 or 4 cloves garlic (or
more)
3 or 4 red hot chilies or any
form of hot pepper, fresh
or dried
3 tbsp fresh grated ginger

Directions

1. Mix a brine of 4 cups (1 liter) water and 4 tbsp salt.
2. Chop cabbage, radish, leeks, and carrots and soak in brine for a few hours or overnight using a plate or a glass bottle filled with water to hold veggies down below surface.
3. Make a spice paste using a microplane grater for garlic and ginger. I used a coffee grinder for the dried chili peppers, removing seeds. Mix spices into a paste.
4. Drain off brine, reserving to the side.
5. Mix spice paste well into vegetables.
6. Stuff into large jar. I used a 2 qt canning jar. Pack down until brine rises. If needed, add

reserve brine so when weighted down the veggies are submerged. Cover top with cloth or paper towel so as to keep bugs out but allow it to breathe.

7. Ferment in warm place for about a week, tasting before moving to fridge.

BISCOTTI

This is a crispy dessert that goes well with a nut mylk, such as our almond mylk recipe (page 121). Keep in a closed container and redehydrate if needed.

Ingredients

3 cups almond flour
1 cup nut mylk or water
1/2 cup raisins, soaked
1/4 cup goji berries, soaked

3 tbsp flaxseed, ground
2 tsp cinnamon powder
1 tsp Celtic Sea Salt

Directions

1. In a bowl, mix almond flour, ground flaxseeds, cinnamon, and salt.
2. Add soak water from raisins and goji berries first and allow the dry batter to absorb liquid for a few minutes.
3. Then add nut mylk or additional water as needed to achieve a consistency in which the batter holds together.

4. Form into loaves about 1–inch high and slice into 1/2–inch pieces.
5. Lay slices on mesh screens and dehydrate at 145 degrees for 2 to 3 hours and then 115 degrees for 2 hours or until crispy.

CHOCOLATE BLISS BALLS

One of our easiest to prepare and most satisfying foods. I have yet to *not* hear an audible "Mmmm!" on first bite. It will be hard to believe that this is raw vegan. Given this, you'll no doubt have to keep them on hand at all times. This form of chocolate does let you have your cake and eat it, too!

Ingredients

1 cup walnuts
1 cup dates

1 cup cacao beans
1/8 cup shredded coconut

Directions

1. Soak walnuts and dates for 1 hour in water.
2. Drain walnuts.
3. Drain dates, reserving soak water.
4. Grind cacao in a blender or coffee grinder.
5. Process all ingredients in a food processor, adding date soak water if needed, until well mixed and firm.
6. Form mixture into balls and freeze for 2 to 3 hours.

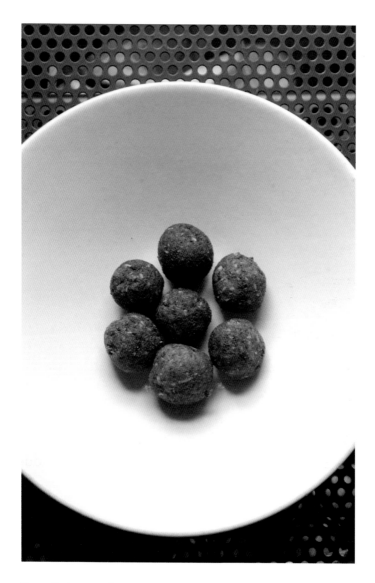

CAULIFLOWER CRUMBLE

This forms the base for many uses, including our herbed cauliflower mash (page 109), as well as couscous and variants. Use as a "grain" and serve with salads or kimchi, etc.

Ingredients

1 head of cauliflower, florets only

Directions

Process cauliflower in a food processor until fully broken up into couscous-like texture.

DAHL

A variant of traditional Indian cabbage dahl. Goes well with our aloo paleek (page 90).

Ingredients

1 handful string beans
1 cup coconut pulp
1/2 cup coconut water
1 tomato
2 tbsp olive oil
2 tsp sea salt

1 clove garlic, minced
1 tsp cumin
1 tsp turmeric
1/4 tsp cayenne pepper
1/4 tsp coriander
1/4 tsp kalonji (black seed)

Directions

1. Blend 2 string beans with the other ingredients in a blender until smooth.
2. Chop remaining string beans into 2–inch pieces.
3. Combine in a mixing bowl with sauce and mix thoroughly.

DATE NUT BARS

Very easy to make and good for food on the go.

Ingredients

10 dates, pitted
5 prunes
1/2 cup walnuts

1/2 tsp vanilla extract
1/4 tsp cinnamon

Directions

1. Soak prunes for 4 hours.
2. Soak dates and walnuts for 1 hour.
3. Drain fruits and nuts, reserving fruit soak water.
4. Blend all ingredients in a food processor.
5. Add fruit soak water if needed for consistency.
6. Spoon out onto cooking sheets and form into bars.
7. Dehydrate at 115 degrees for 1 hour.
8. Flip over onto mesh and continue dehydrating for 1 hour.

EGGPLANT MARINADE

An excellent addition to tortillas stuffed with sprouts and pâté.

Ingredients

2 eggplants
1/2 cup olive oil
1/2 cup lemon juice

2 tsp herbes de Provence
1/4 tsp sea salt

Directions

1. De-skin the eggplants.
2. Slice eggplant into very thin medallions.
3. Mix all ingredients in a bowl, massaging the eggplant with the marinade.
4. Allow to sit in marinade for 4 hours or more.

FALAFEL BALLS

When I discovered that this was possible, fried falafels were forever off my wish list. You will want to eat them as soon as they pop out of the dehydrator, warm and crispy. If storing, redehydrate for 10 to 20 minutes for desired crispiness, as the moisture from the inner core will make the outside soft again. The balance of crispiness and softness is dependent on eating soon after dehydrating.

Ingredients

2 cups sprouted chickpeas
1 cup soaked sunflower
   seeds
2 garlic cloves
1/4 cup olive oil
1 cup leeks

1 lemon juiced
2 cups cilantro
2 tbsp Global South
   Seasoning Mix (see our
   recipe, page 65)

Directions

Sprouting chickpeas: (1/2 cup dry chickpeas yields 2 cups sprouted chickpeas)

1. Soak dry chickpeas in water for 12 hours.
2. Drain.
3. Rinse chickpeas 2 to 3 times daily. Give the soak water to your houseplants—they will love it!
4. Sprout chickpeas for 3 days, making sure they get air and are in the dark or semidark.
5. Before adding to food processor, boil water and pour over sprouted chickpeas. This converts the starches to complex carbohydrates.

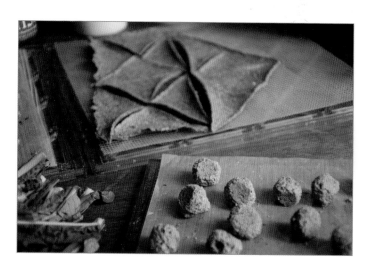

To make falafel balls:

1. Combine all ingredients in a food processor and process until well blended.
2. Process all ingredients in food processor with S-blade.
3. Roll mash into ping-pong–sized balls.
4. Place on teflex sheets in dehydrator.
5. Dehydrate at 145 degrees for 2 hours.
6. Remove from teflex sheets and dehydrate on mesh sheets at 145 degrees for 4 hours or until desired crispiness is achieved.

FRED'S ALMOND DELIGHT

This is a delicious, crowd-pleasing, and easy-to-make dessert.

Reuse the food-processed raw almonds (or other nuts) from the recipe for nut mylks (page 121) after the mylk has been strained and what remains are the finely chopped nuts. In a mixing bowl, stir with honey and maple syrup (equal parts of each to a total combined amount of 1/3 the nut residue). Add cinnamon and nutmeg in large quantities.

By reusing the processed raw nuts instead of discarding or composting them, you have created a delicious dessert! Serve chilled. Can be refrigerated in sealed container for 5 days.

GLOBAL SOUTH SEASONING MIX

For use with falafel balls.

Ingredients

2 tbsp paprika
1 tbsp oregano
1 tbsp coriander
1 tbsp sea salt

2 tsp cumin
1 tsp black pepper
1 tsp cayenne pepper
1 tbsp kalonji (black seed)

GREEN GREENER GREENEST JUICES

In a vertical high-speed juicer (not a blender or a food processor) with a large mouth opening, juice a variety of sturdy and hard green leafy vegetables (such as kale, celery, bok choy, etc.) with cucumber, ginger, and parsley. Add fruits for a more sweetened taste. Your entire house will smell like a vegetable garden. The juice can be refrigerated or even frozen. Serve cold or with ice cubes.

HARD-BOILED EGG

The simplest of all our recipes, with endless applications in salads or tortillas. The sulfur in black salt provides the "egg" flavor.

Ingredients

1 ripe avocado
1/2 tsp black salt

Directions

Mash avocado with salt.

HERBED CAULIFLOWER MASH

You will not miss mashed potatoes after trying this. Both pine nuts and macadamias create a very creamy flavor, taking the place of butter in traditional mashed potatoes. Sunflower seeds could replace pine nuts, as pine nuts are expensive.

Ingredients

1 cup cauliflower crumble
1 cup pine nuts
1/2 cup macadamia nuts
5 tbsp olive oil
2 tbsp herbes de Provence

1/2 tbsp minced garlic
1/2 tsp Celtic Sea Salt
1/4 tsp ground black
   pepper

Directions

Process all ingredients in a food processor, adding a small amount of water to achieve smoothness.

INDIAN FLAT BREAD

Wheat- and yeast-free . . . who says bread can't be raw? Serve with dahl (page 99), topped with our just like butter (page 112).

Ingredients

1 head cauliflower
1 carrot
1 red bell pepper
2 cups flaxseeds
1 cup soaked sunflower
   seeds

1 1/2 cups water
2 tsp turmeric
1 tsp cumin
1 tsp cinnamon
1 tsp sea salt

Directions

1. Chop up cauliflower, carrot, and red bell pepper, and then process in a food processor with the S-blade.
2. In a bowl, mix all ingredients well.
3. Spread batter onto teflex sheets evenly to a thickness of 1/4 inch.
4. Dehydrate at 145 degrees for 1 hour.
5. Flip over, removing teflex sheets, and continue to dehydrate for 2 hours.

Raw Extreme Manifesto

JALAPENO SAUCE

This is an extraordinarily zesty hot sauce.

Ingredients

2–3 lbs of firm jalapeno peppers, de-stemmed
2 cups olive oil (need not be extra virgin—may substitute vegetable oil or any oil, such as butternut squash, sunflower seed, etc.)
1 cup white vinegar
2 tbsp salt

Directions

Blend ingredients together until creamy. Use as a dip or hot sauce with a variety of dishes.

JUST LIKE BUTTER

Simple, nondairy, no soy, nonhydrogenated, richly nutritious. This will change your ideas about traditional butter or margarine.

Ingredients

1/2 cup coconut oil
2 cups coconut pulp
1 1/2 lemons

1/2 cup flax oil
1 tsp sea salt

Directions

1. Peel the lemons and de-seed.
2. Blend all ingredients until smooth and creamy.

KALE CHIPS TO DIE FOR

For a small dehydrator, use 10 stalks of kale.

Ingredients

2 cups oil (extra virgin, butternut squash, or grapeseed)

1 cup Bragg's amino acid

3 tbsp dried curry powder

Directions

1. Strip kale leaves from stalks (save the stalks as they can be juiced later).

2. Make marinade (in mixing bowl, combine oil, Braggs liquid amino acid, and dried curry powder; whisk until blended).

3. Stir stripped kale leaves in marinade and let sit for 30 minutes, making sure all kale leaves are saturated with the marinade mix.

4. Using a dehydrator sheet, spread the marinated kale leaves on each tray sheet; slightly touching is fine, but don't overlap.

5. Insert tray sheets into dehydrator shelving slots.

6. Cover the dehydrator and set to run for 3.5 to 4 hours at 115 degrees (as the kale leaves dehydrate, you'll smell the delicious aroma).

7. After 3.5 to 4 hours, take out the trays and remove the dehydrated kale chips into a serving bowl.

8. Dehydrated kale chips should not be refrigerated at all but kept in a serving bowl for a meal or snacking.

KEY LIME PIE

Amazingly quick and easy to make. Treat yourself and friends to a dessert delight with an extremely low glycemic index.

Ingredients for the Crust

2 cups soaked pecans
1/4 tsp nutmeg
1/4 tsp cinnamon
1/4 tsp black pepper
1/4 tsp sea salt

Directions

1. Process all ingredients in a food processor with the S-blade until it thickens into a ball.
2. Press evenly into a pie plate and chill.

Ingredients for the Filling

1/2 avocado
1/2 cup coconut water
pulp from the coconut
4 tbsp lemon juice
4 tbsp lime juice
1/2 vanilla bean or 1 tsp
   vanilla extract
1/2 tsp sea salt
1/4 tsp stevia or 2 tbsp
   agave nectar
1 tsp psyllium husks

Directions

1. In a blender, process all except the psyllium until creamy.
2. Pour into a bowl, add psyllium, and mix well.
3. Add to pie crust, smoothing out to the edges.
4. Chill in refrigerator for 1 to 2 hours.

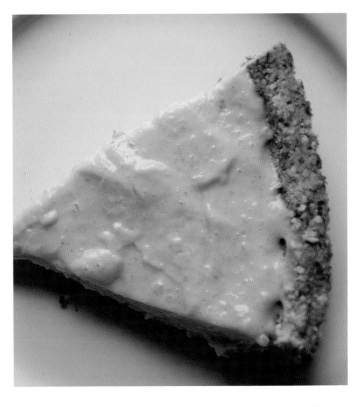

LEMON DILL DRESSING

A sharp and creamy salad dressing.

Ingredients

1/2 cup olive oil
1/2 cup lemon juice
1 tbsp tahini

2 tsp dill
1/2 tsp Celtic Sea Salt

Directions

Blend all ingredients until creamy.

MACADAMIA NUT CHEESE

Great with our sun-dried tomato flax crackers (page 133) or in a tortilla with salad greens or just as a snack.

Ingredients

4 cups macadamia nuts
1/2 cup lemon juice
2 tbsp nutritional yeast

1 green onion
2 tsp sea salt

Directions

1. Soak the nuts for 1 hour.
2. Dice the onion, using the white and 1 or 2 inches of the green.
3. Process in a food processor using the S-blade.
4. Spoon blobs of the mix onto teflex sheets.
5. Dehydrate at 115 degrees for 4 to 6 hours.

MEDITERRANEAN SALAD

A classic nonleafy salad.

Ingredients

Large chopped pieces of tomato

Large chopped pieces of cucumber

Small chopped pieces of red onion

1 cup fine chopped parsley

Extra virgin olive oil drizzled heavily upon above

Salt, pepper and cumin to taste

Directions

Mix and stir well. Serve chilled after leaving in refrigerator 1 hour.

NUT AND FRUIT BAR

Another variant on snack food to go. Chia seeds provide meganutrition and, together with the prunes, great fiber.

Ingredients:

1 cup dried prunes
1 cup Brazil nuts
1/2 cup hemp seeds
1/2 cup goji berries

1/2 cup Thompson raisins
1 tsp chia seeds
1 tsp grated ginger

Directions

1. Soak prunes and Brazil nuts separately in water, 8 hours or overnight.
2. Soak goji berries 1 to 2 hours.
3. Drain Brazil nuts only.
4. Combine all ingredients, including the water used for soaking goji and prunes, in a food processor and blend.
5. Form mash into rectangular bars.
6. Place on teflex sheets and dehydrate at 100 degrees for 4 hours.

NUT MYLKS

(I use this spelling to distance nut milks from animal milks.)

Nut mylks allow you to get good fats without a lot of work in digesting. They will keep only for a day, so drink them fresh. Among the nuts and seeds that make delicious mylk are sunflower seeds, almonds, macadamias, Brazil, pumpkin, sesame, pecans, and walnuts.

Please see directions on the following page.

Germination Chart

SEED TYPE	DRY MEASURE	SOAKING TIME	YIELD
almonds	1 cup	12 hours	1 cup
pecans	1 cup	1–2 hours	1 cup
walnuts	1 cup	1–2 hours	1 cup
macadamia		do not soak	
pine nuts		do not soak	
Brazil nuts		do not soak	
hulled pumpkin seeds	1 cup	4 hours	2 cups
hulled sunflower seeds	1 cup	4 hours	2.5 cups
hulled white sesame seeds	1 cup	4 hours	1 cup
flax seeds	1 cup seed	8 hours	1 cup
flax seeds for grinding		do not soak	

Ingredients

1 cup nuts or seeds
2–3 cups water

2 tbsp lecithin

Directions

1. Soak nuts according to germination chart.
2. Drain and rinse.
3. In a blender, add nuts to the 2 to 3 cups water and blend on high speed for 1 minute.
4. Using a nut mylk bag, cheesecloth, or loose weave muslin fabric, strain and squeeze out liquid into a container.
5. Pour mylk back into blender, add lecithin, and blend lightly. The lecithin will act as a binder to help keep the mylk from separating.

Experiment with variations of flavoring the mylk. Almond Chai is one of our favorites.

NUT MYLKS: ALMOND CHAI

Ingredients

3 cups almond mylk
3 tbsp raw cacao powder
1 tbsp ginger juice
1 tbsp cinnamon

1 tbsp nutmeg
1 tsp cardamom
1/2 tsp stevia

Directions

Blend all ingredients in a blender and serve chilled.

ONION BHAJIS

Once again, no need for deep frying. These are a crowd-pleaser. It's hard to stop at just one.

Ingredients

1 cup sunflower seeds, soaked
1 cup walnuts, soaked
2 cups red onions
2 tsp paprika
1/4 tsp cayenne pepper

2 cloves garlic
1 bunch cilantro
1 red pepper, de-seeded
1 tsp kalonji (black seed)
1 tsp cumin
3 tbsp olive oil

Directions

1. Finely chop red onions and garlic.
2. Chop red pepper and cilantro.
3. Process all ingredients except 1 cup red onions in a food processor using the S-blade.
4. In a bowl, add mixture to remaining onions.
5. Form batter into balls a bit smaller than ping-pong balls.
6. Dehydrate on teflex sheets at 135 degrees for 1 or 2 hours.
7. Remove teflex and continue to dehydrate on mesh for 4 to 6 hours. Balls should be a bit crispy on the outside and soft inside.

PURPLE KALE CHEESE CHIPS

One of the world's healthiest "chips." These don't need any dips to enjoy. Just inhale.

Ingredients

1 bunch purple kale
1 cup soaked sunflower
  seeds
1 lemon, juiced
1 red bell pepper

2 tbsp ume plum vinegar
2 tbsp miso
2 tbsp olive oil
2 tbsp Global South
  Seasoning Mix

Directions

1. De-stem kale.
2. In a food processor, add other ingredients and process until creamy.
3. In a large mixing bowl, massage paste into kale leaves.
4. Place kale on teflex sheets.
5. Dehydrate at 115 degrees for 3 hours or until crispy.

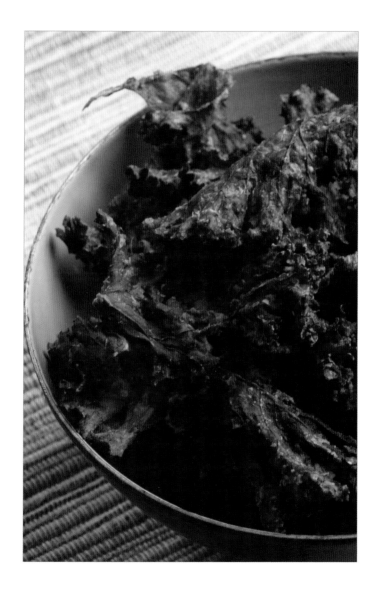

PERSIMMON PUDDING

Persimmons, so delicious on their own, are only slightly modified here, adding the power of chia seeds as a complement. Chia seed benefits are numerous. They have the highest known level of omega-3 alpha-linoleic acid, more than double that of fish oils, and a balance of omega-6, another of the essential fatty acids. They provide an incredible blend of protein, fiber, complex carbohydrates, and antioxidants, resulting in higher levels of available energy.

Ingredients

2 ripe persimmons
1 tsp chia seeds

Directions

1. Blend ingredients in a blender.
2. Chill in fridge for 1 hour.

QUINOA CRACKERS

These crackers are crisper than our other flax crackers due to the sprouted quinoa. Sprouting grains is the only way to make them digestible raw, releasing enzyme inhibitors and making them live.

Ingredients

1 cup sprouted quinoa
1 cup flaxseeds, soaked
2 tbsp chia seeds
1/2 red bell pepper

1/2 tsp ground black
  pepper
1/2 tsp kalonji (black seed)
1/2 tsp Celtic Sea Salt

Directions

1. Process all ingredients in a food processor.
2. Spread batter onto teflex sheets, 1/4–inch thick, into one rectangle per sheet.
3. Dehydrate at 145 degrees for 2 to 3 hours.
4. Turn over onto mesh screens, removing teflex, and continue to dehydrate at 115 degrees for 5 hours or until crisp.

To sprout quinoa, soak 1 cup quinoa in water for 3 hours, drain water, and then let sit in open container for 24 hours in semidarkness. Rinse again before using.

RED PEPPER CURRY DRESSING

Ingredients

1 cup red bell pepper
1/4 cup olive oil
2 tbsp lemon juice

1 tbsp curry powder
1/2 tbsp sea salt

Directions

Blend all ingredients until creamy.

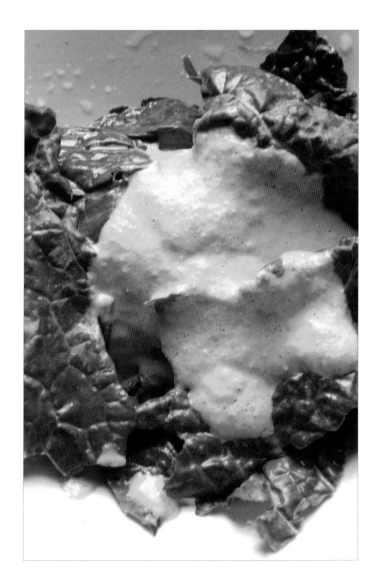

SASHIMI PLATTER AND DIP

Ingredients

Assorted sliced raw fish (tuna, hamachi or yellowtail, salmon de-skinned, mackerel, swordfish . . . actually any edible saltwater or freshwater fish will be fine)

Bragg Liquid Aminos protein substitute for soy sauce
Chili oil
Sesame oil
Thinly sliced fresh or pickled ginger
Finely chopped scallions

Directions

1. Combine equal parts Bragg liquid, chili, and sesame oil and put in dipping bowl.
2. Garnish the raw fish with the fine chopped scallions.
3. Use the ginger as a condiment.
4. Dip sliced raw fish in the sauce and eat.

SUN-DRIED TOMATO FLAX CRACKERS

Serve with our xtremely compassionate foie gras (page 144) or on their own. Flaxseeds provide healthy fiber and omega-3, -6 and -9 fatty acids in a fresh form, which is better than extracted in oil form. Power to the immune system! One can also grind flax and sprinkle on salads for added nutrition, flavor, and texture. The more the better!

Ingredients

1 cup sun-dried tomatoes
2 cups flaxseeds
1/4 cup chopped parsley
1/2 tsp oregano
1/2 tsp thyme

1/2 tsp sage
1 tbsp olive oil
1/2 tsp sea salt
1/2 tsp cayenne pepper

Directions

1. Soak sun-dried tomatoes for 3 to 4 hours.
2. Soak flaxseeds in 2 cups water for 8 hours.
3. Blend sun-dried tomatoes and parsley.
4. Mix all ingredients in a mixing bowl.

5. Spread mix onto teflex sheets in a rectangle, 1/4 inch thick or less on each sheet.
6. With a butter knife, cut a rectangular grid through the spread.
7. Dehydrate at 145 degrees for 2 to 3 hours.
8. Turn over and dehydrate on mesh sheets for 8 to 10 hours at 115 degrees.

TAHINI

This is the raw version of tahini, normally sold in cooked form. As all of these recipes demonstrate, there's no reason to cook most food if it can be had raw, leaving intact the enzymes and nutrients. Great as a salad dressing and with falafel.

Ingredients

2 cups white sesame seeds
1 cup water (for blending)
1/2 cup lemon juice

1 1/2 tsp sea salt
1 garlic clove, minced

Directions

1. Soak sesame seeds for 4 hours.
2. Drain and rinse.
3. Blend all ingredients until creamy.

TORTILLAS

It will astound you that a raw bread can be as flexible and versatile as this one. Stuff these with any salad mix, pâté, bhajis, or falafel balls.

Ingredients

1 cup golden flaxseeds
1/2 ripe avocado
1/4 cup celery
1/4 cup cilantro

1 tsp turmeric
1 tsp sea salt
1 tbsp apple cider vinegar
2 cups water

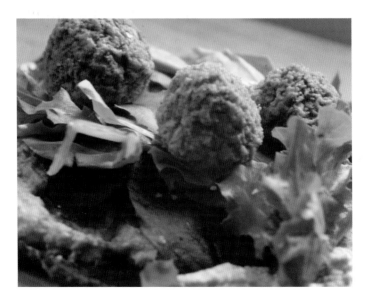

Directions

1. Grind flaxseeds in Vitamix blender and set aside.
2. Blend celery, cilantro, and avocado in a food processor.
3. Add remaining ingredients except flax and blend.
4. Add flax to mix and blend. The consistency should be a bit thicker than pancake mix.
5. Spread mix on teflex sheets to about 1/4-inch thick and 6 inches in diameter.
6. Dehydrate at 95 degrees for 2 to 3 hours; flip over onto mesh and dehydrate for 2 to 3 hours more.
7. Check after 2 hours for pliability. They should still be soft, not brittle.

UDON NOODLE SOUP

Once again, the raw version puts to shame the needless application of destructive heat to the cooked version. The rich and complex blend of spices and fats from the coconut pulp make this an exhilarating soup.

Ingredients

3 cups coconut water
1 tbsp lemongrass, finely chopped
1 tbsp grated ginger
1 garlic clove
5 Kaffir lime leaves
1 cup coconut pulp
1/2 cup snow peas

1/2 cup red bell pepper, deseeded and julienned
1 stalk green onion
1/2 tbsp amino acids or wheat-free tamari
1 tsp sesame oil
1/2 tsp ume plum vinegar

Directions

1. Chop garlic.
2. Blend coconut water, garlic, ginger, lemongrass, and lime leaves until smooth.
3. Strain through a fine mesh strainer into a bowl and discard the pulp.

4. Slice coconut pulp into thin strips the width of udon noodles, about 1/4 inch.
5. Add remaining ingredients to soup.
6. Garnish servings with scallions. This will serve four.

VEGETABLE TEMPURA

"Fried" never tasted so clean! Incredibly savory!

Ingredients

2 cups broccoli florets
2 cups cauliflower florets
1 cup zucchini, sliced into
   disks
1/2 cup pistachios,
   unsoaked
1 cup sunflower seeds,
   soaked

1/2 cup lemon juice
3 tsp sea salt
1/2 cup olive oil
1 tsp coriander
2 tsp cumin
1 tsp kalonji (black seed)
1/4 tsp cayenne pepper
1 cup water

Directions

1. Blend nuts, lemon juice, spices, salt, and olive oil in a blender, adding water until it is smooth.
2. Combine with the vegetables in a mixing bowl and toss together with hands until all the vegetables are coated.
3. Place mixture onto teflex sheets and dehydrate at 145 degrees for 2 hours.

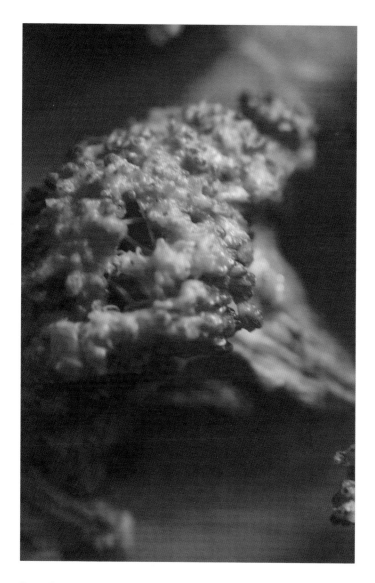

WALNUTS, CASHEWS, NUTS, AND SEEDS ... OH, MY!

Raw nuts and seeds can be mixed with dried fruit to provide a quick and easy trail mix that can last for a very long time without refrigeration and be carried on trips as a snack.

WATERMELON AND FROZEN BLUEBERRY SMOOTHIE

Our favorite summertime smoothie! This is a truly energizing and light liquid food that will keep your hunger at bay for a long time due to the power of chia seeds and maca root powder, both said to be the food of indigenous warriors going to battle! This tonic will immediately provide palpable hydration and energy.

Ingredients

3 cups watermelon pulp
1/2 cup frozen blueberries
2 tbsp chia seeds
1 tbsp maca root powder
2 tsp ginger juice

1 tbsp apple cider vinegar
juice from watermelon rind
(as much or as little as
you need)

Directions

Blend all ingredients in a blender.

XTREMELY COMPASSIONATE FOIE GRAS

Quite honestly, this tastes a lot better than "real" foie gras, the engorged liver of force-fed ducks. It is truly absurd that the products of such practices are considered "delicacies." This pâté will give one a much higher frequency, indeed, of revolutionary proportions, of delicacy and delight. Talk about alienated labor!

Ingredients

1 cup sprouted red lentils
1 cup soaked walnuts
1/2 red onion
1/4 cup olive oil
1 tbsp Bragg Liquid Aminos

1 tbsp mirin
2 tsp ume plum vinegar
2 tbsp miso
1 tsp black pepper

Directions

1. How to sprout lentils: Soak lentils in water for 8 hours. (See falafel balls recipe on page 102 for the procedure to sprout chick peas and follow the

same steps; (1/4 cup dry lentils yields about 1 cup sprouted lentils.)

2. Soak walnuts 1 to 2 hours and drain.
3. Combine all ingredients in a food processor and process until creamy.

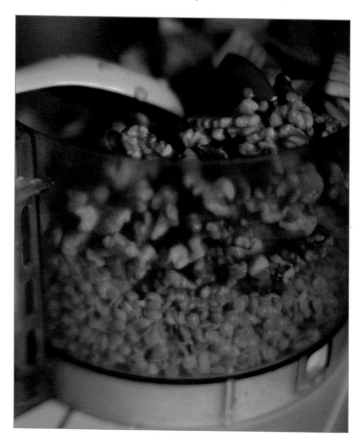

YAM CHIPS

These chips store and travel well. I like the sweet yams best.

Ingredients

4 cups yams, sliced
1/2 cup olive oil
2 tbsp sea salt

1 tsp black pepper, ground
2 tsp lime juice

Directions

1. Slice yam with a mandoline or spiralizer or food processor using the chipping blade.
2. Combine all ingredients in a bowl and massage until all chips are coated.
3. Dehydrate chips on mesh screens at 145 degrees for 2 hours and then at 115 degrees for another 2 hours or until desired crispiness is achieved.

YOUR BASIC SALAD

All sorts of leafy greens (including Asian greens), herbs, basil leaves, red onion, cucumbers, carrots, and a wide assortment of raw fruits and vegetables, including dried fruits, can be tossed and mixed as a salad. For a simple and easy dressing, try extra virgin olive oil and vinegar. Sprouts, avocado slices, chopped scallions, or seeds can top it off.

ZUCCHINI NOODLES WITH PESTO

Any squash can be used—yellow, butternut. For crunchier texture, try daikon, carrot, or jicama.

Pesto Ingredients

2 cups fresh cilantro
1 cup fresh basil
1 cup walnuts
3/4 cup olive oil
2 tbsp lemon juice

2 tbsp sage
3 garlic cloves
2 tsp Celtic Sea Salt
1/2 tsp cayenne pepper

Pesto Directions

Process all ingredients in a food processor with S-blade until creamy.

Noodle Ingredients

3 zucchini

Noodle Directions

With a spiralizer, process zucchini into noodles. Mix 3/4 cup pesto with noodles.

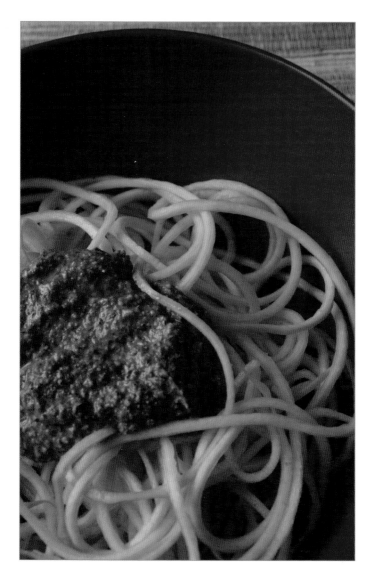

ZUCCHINI BREAD

A dense and hearty bread, a bit like manna or fruit bread.

Ingredients

2 cups walnuts, soaked
1/2 cup raisins, soaked
1/4 cup goji berries, soaked
1 cup zucchini
1 1/4 cup flaxseeds, ground

2 tsp cinnamon
1/2 tsp nutmeg
1/2 vanilla bean
1 tsp Celtic Sea Salt

Directions

1. Blend raisins, zucchini, and vanilla bean using raisin soak water.
2. Chop up walnuts in a food processor with the S-blade.
3. Grind flaxseeds in a blender.
4. Mix all ingredients in a bowl, adding goji berries and spices.
5. Form 2 loaves and slice into 1/2-inch pieces.
6. Dehydrate at 145 degrees for 2 to 3 hours and then 115 for 2 hours, checking for desired level of moisture.

INDEX